EVERYTHING YOU NEED TO START AFIB DIET COOKBOOK FOR BEGINNERS

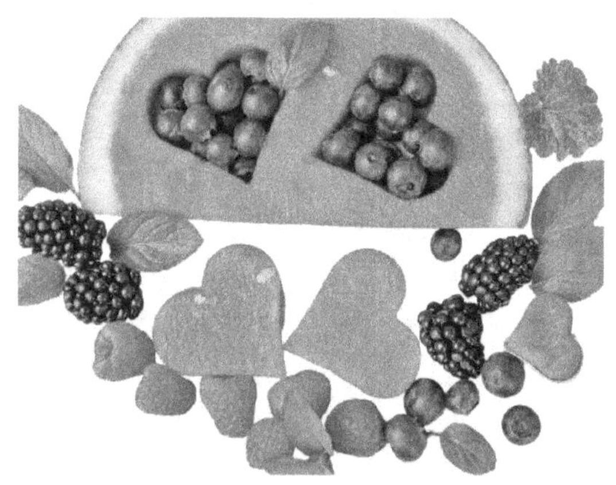

Nourishing and Wholesome Culinary Recipes to Naturally Address Atrial Fibrillation, Heart Disease, Stroke, Fatigue, and Combat Obesity.

Felicia O. Pace

Table of Contents

"Unlocking a Healthier Heart Rhythm: Your Journey to a Vibrant Life Begins Here"

Welcome to a transformative journey toward a healthier, more vibrant life! In the hustle and bustle of our daily lives, health often takes a backseat, and for those navigating the challenges of Atrial Fibrillation (AFib), this journey becomes even more complex. As your expert guide, writing coach, and companion on this path, I'm thrilled to introduce you to the *"AFib Diet Cookbook for Beginners."*

In the symphony of life, our heart plays the lead role, orchestrating the rhythm that propels us forward. But what happens when that rhythm falters, when the heart's tune becomes irregular, echoing the challenges of Atrial Fibrillation? Fear not, for within the pages of this cookbook lies a powerful key – a culinary journey tailored to bring harmony to your heart.

I understand the intricate dance of emotions that accompanies an AFib diagnosis. As a seasoned cardiologist, nutritional expert, and chef, my life's work has been dedicated to unraveling the complexities of heart health. Through years of clinical practice and culinary exploration, I've witnessed the transformative impact of a diet designed specifically for those grappling with AFib.

Why an AFib Diet Cookbook? Because every morsel you consume holds the potential to be a healing note in your heart's melody. This cookbook is not just about recipes; it's a lifeline, a compass guiding you towards foods that nourish, strengthen, and soothe your heart.

Within these pages, you'll discover more than just delicious recipes; you'll find a roadmap to reclaiming control over your health. This isn't just a cookbook; it's a comprehensive guide crafted to empower beginners on their AFib journey.

We'll embark on this culinary adventure in ten enriching chapters. From unraveling the intricacies of AFib and understanding its connection to diet, to exploring the science behind heart-healthy nutrition, stocking your kitchen with essential ingredients, and crafting delectable breakfasts, lunches, dinners, snacks, and desserts – this book is a holistic guide.

But, dear reader, I won't reveal it all here. Picture tantalizing recipes, each a fusion of health and flavor. Envision your kitchen becoming a haven of heart-healthy creations. Anticipate the joy of nurturing your heart, not just physically but emotionally through the act of cooking.

Now, you might wonder – can I really master this? Fear not, for I'm your personal culinary coach, offering not just recipes but guidance, tips, and the assurance that each step is tailored for beginners. Your journey is our shared success, and every hurdle you face, consider it conquered with knowledge and flavor.

So, are you ready to embark on a culinary expedition that promises not just nourishment but a symphony of flavors tailored for your heart? The "AFib Diet Cookbook for Beginners" is more than a book; it's your ally, and together, we're about to create a masterpiece – a life well-lived, heart well-loved. Let the journey begin

Understanding AFib

"Decoding the Rhythms: Mastering the Basics of Atrial Fibrillation"

Hello, fellow travelers on the road to a healthier heart! It's wonderful to have you join us for a closer look at Atrial Fibrillation (AFib). No need to worry if the term sounds a bit technical; think of it as getting to know your heart's unique dance moves, and we're here to make it as simple as your favorite recipe.

Demystifying AFib: Your Heart's Dance Partner

Picture your heart as the star of the show, gracefully leading the dance of life. Now, imagine AFib as the unexpected dance partner throwing in some unexpected moves. Together, we're going to unravel why this uninvited guest showed up and how to help your heart reclaim its smooth groove.

Identifying the Dance Floor Troublemakers: Unmasking AFib Triggers

Ever wonder what makes your heart trip over its own steps? It could be stress, a sneaky extra cup of coffee, or even that bag of chips. In this chapter, we're pulling back the curtain to reveal these sneaky culprits, empowering you to regain control over the rhythm of your heart.

Listening to Your Heart's Whisper: Recognizing AFib's Subtle Signals

AFib doesn't always make a grand entrance; it prefers a subtle whisper. Imagine your heart trying to tell you something important, but in a hushed tone. We're going to explore these gentle signals – the skips, the flutters – so you can tune in and truly understand what your heart is saying.

Nutrition as Your Heart's Conductor: The Power of Diet in AFib Management
Now, let's talk about food – the unsung hero in this heartwarming tale. Your meals can be the maestro, orchestrating a beautiful rhythm in your heart's dance. We'll bridge the gap between what's on your plate and the beast within, unveiling the incredible influence of nutrition on managing AFib.

Unlocking the Nutrition-Heart Harmony
Get ready to be amazed as we unravel the special connection between your food choices and your heart's dance. It's not just about eating; it's about understanding the language your heart speaks through your meals. Your diet becomes the translator, turning the whispers into a beautiful, harmonious conversation.

The Science of Nutrition and Heart Health

Hook: "Fueling Your Heart: Unveiling the Power of Nutrient-rich Foods"
oin me as we transform nutritional insights into practical, heartwarming wisdom for your AFib Diet Cookbook journey.

Essential Nutrients: Your Heart's Trusty Companions

Think of these nutrients not just as superheroes but as your heart's most trusted friends. Picture vitamin C as the defender of your immune system, omega-3 fatty acids as the guardians of your blood vessels – a team working together to keep your heart strong. By bringing these nutrients to life, we turn them into allies, making your meals a powerful force for your heart's well-being.

Your Plate, Your Heart: Crafting a Culinary Love Affair

Your plate is more than just a source of nutrition; it's a love letter to your heart. Let's infuse emotion into this relationship. Imagine each meal as a heartfelt gesture, a way of showing love and care to your heart. Your plate becomes a trusted companion, delivering a comforting embrace with every wholesome bite. This emotional connection makes your dietary choices a journey of love and health.

The Dance of Food and Heart: A Beautiful Symphony Simplified

The dance floor metaphor is charming, but let's simplify the chemistry between food and heart rhythm even further. Visualize your heart as a conductor and each nutrient as a musician playing a unique role in the symphony of your health. This simple image transforms complex processes into a relatable story, making it easier for beginners to grasp.

Backed by Science: Turning Studies into Everyday Wisdom
Rather than just mentioning scientific studies, let's make them a seamless part of the conversation. After discussing the importance of omega-3 fatty acids, share a snippet of a study that highlights their real-world benefits. This way, we're not just talking facts; we're showing how these nutritional insights apply to your daily life, making science relatable and practical.

Your Culinary Adventure Begins: A Journey of Self-Discovery
Now, it's not just about following recipes; it's about embarking on a journey of self-discovery. Your kitchen is the stage, and you are the protagonist. The AFib Diet Cookbook isn't just a guide; it's a companion on your adventure to a healthier and happier you.

"Transforming Your Pantry: Setting the Stage for a Heartwarming Culinary Adventure"

Mastering the Grocery Store: A Heart-Healthy Adventure

Imagine strolling through the grocery store like a seasoned explorer, with a shopping list tailored just for you and your heart. We're talking about fruits that practically shout, "I'm packed with nutrients!" and veggies that do a little dance when you pick them up. No complicated guides here – just practical tips for a stress-free, heart-healthy grocery shopping experience.

Cracking the Code on Food Labels: Your Superpower Unleashed

Ever feel like food labels are trying to play hide-and-seek with the good stuff? Together, we'll decode the mysteries. I'll share some simple tricks to read labels like a pro, helping you distinguish between the heart-boosting champs and the sneaky ingredients you might want to avoid. No secret handshakes needed – just straightforward guidance.

Fresh vs. Frozen: The Battle of the Goodies
Let's settle the fresh vs. frozen debate, shall we? I'll be your referee, guiding you through the advantages and disadvantages of each. No need for a culinary degree; just some practical insights to help you decide which goodies are best for your heart and your taste buds.

Spices, Herbs, and Flavorful Magic: Because Healthy Shouldn't Mean Bland
In our heart-healthy kitchen, flavor is the secret ingredient. We're diving into the world of spices and herbs that will turn your meals into a taste sensation. Say goodbye to the misconception that healthy eating is synonymous with blandness. I'll show you how to spice things up without compromising your heart health.

Smart Choices on a Budget: Nourishing Your Heart Without Breaking the Bank
Eating well doesn't mean waving goodbye to your hard-earned cash. I've got some savvy tips on finding heart-healthy ingredients that won't make your wallet do a disappearing act. It's about making choices that align with your health goals without feeling like you need a financial advisor.

Your Basket, Your Heart: Making Mindful Choices

As you fill your basket, remember, you're not just shopping for groceries; you're investing in your heart's well-being. I'll help you make choices that suit your lifestyle and health aspirations. This isn't about restrictions – it's about giving yourself the power to make mindful decisions that feel right for you.

CHAPTER 2

Breakfast

"Rise and Shine: A Symphony of Flavors to Kickstart Your Heart"

Berry Bliss Smoothie Bowl
Ingredients: Mixed berries, Greek yogurt, chia seeds, honey.
Preparation: Blend berries and yogurt, top with chia seeds and a drizzle of honey.
Prep Time: 5 minutes.

Avocado Toast with Tomato Salsa
Ingredients: Whole-grain bread, ripe avocado, tomatoes, cilantro.
Preparation: Mash avocado on toast, top with tomato salsa and cilantro.
Prep Time: 10 minutes.

Oatmeal Power Bowl
Ingredients: Rolled oats, almond milk, banana, almonds, cinnamon.
Preparation: Cook oats in almond milk, top with sliced banana, almonds, and a sprinkle of cinnamon.
Prep Time: 15 minutes.

Greek Yogurt Parfait

Ingredients: Greek yogurt, granola, mixed berries, honey.

Preparation: Layer yogurt, granola, and berries, drizzle with honey.

Prep Time: 5 minutes.

Spinach and Feta Omelet

Ingredients: Eggs, spinach, feta cheese, cherry tomatoes.

Preparation: Whisk eggs, add spinach, feta, and tomatoes, cook as an omelet.

Prep Time: 10 minutes.

Whole Grain Pancakes

Ingredients: Whole grain flour, almond milk, eggs, blueberries.

Preparation: Mix ingredients, cook pancakes, top with fresh blueberries.

Prep Time: 20 minutes.

Chia Seed Pudding

Ingredients: Chia seeds, almond milk, vanilla extract, strawberries.

Preparation: Mix chia seeds, almond milk, and vanilla, refrigerate overnight, top with sliced strawberries.

Prep Time: 5 minutes (plus overnight chilling).

Banana Walnut Muffins

Ingredients: Whole wheat flour, ripe bananas, walnuts.

Preparation: Mix ingredients, bake in muffin tin.

Prep Time: 25 minutes.

Sweet Potato Hash

Ingredients: Sweet potatoes, bell peppers, onions, eggs.

Preparation: Sauté veggies, top with eggs, cook until eggs are done.

Prep Time: 15 minutes.

Apple Cinnamon Quinoa Bowl

Ingredients: Quinoa, almond milk, apples, cinnamon.

Preparation: Cook quinoa in almond milk, top with sliced apples and a sprinkle of cinnamon.

Prep Time: 20 minutes.

Peanut Butter Banana Wrap

Ingredients: Whole wheat tortilla, peanut butter, banana.

Preparation: Spread peanut butter on tortilla, add banana slices, wrap it up.

Prep Time: 5 minutes.

Coconut Mango Smoothie

Ingredients: Coconut milk, mango, spinach, banana.

Preparation: Blend ingredients until smooth.

Prep Time: 10 minutes.

Egg and Veggie Breakfast Burrito

Ingredients: Whole grain tortilla, eggs, bell peppers, black beans.

Preparation: Scramble eggs, add veggies, roll into a burrito.

Prep Time: 15 minutes.

Yogurt and Berry Parfait

Ingredients: Yogurt, mixed berries, granola.

Preparation: Layer yogurt, berries, and granola.

Prep Time: 5 minutes.

Almond Butter Overnight Oats

Ingredients: Rolled oats, almond milk, almond butter, banana.

Preparation: Mix ingredients, refrigerate overnight.

Prep Time: 5 minutes (plus overnight chilling).

Cottage Cheese and Pineapple Bowl

Ingredients: Cottage cheese, pineapple chunks.

Preparation: Combine cottage cheese and pineapple.

Prep Time: 5 minutes.

Mushroom and Spinach Scramble

Ingredients: Eggs, mushrooms, spinach, feta cheese.

Preparation: Scramble eggs, add mushrooms, spinach, and feta.

Prep Time: 15 minutes.

Blueberry Almond Smoothie

Ingredients: Almond milk, blueberries, almonds, yogurt.

Preparation: Blend ingredients until smooth.

Prep Time: 10 minutes.

Peach and Pecan Overnight Oats

Ingredients: Rolled oats, almond milk, peaches, pecans.

Preparation: Mix ingredients, refrigerate overnight.

Prep Time: 5 minutes (plus overnight chilling).

Tomato Basil Breakfast Wrap

Ingredients: Whole grain tortilla, eggs, cherry tomatoes, fresh basil.

Preparation: Scramble eggs, add tomatoes and basil, wrap it up.

Prep Time: 10 minutes.

"Midday Euphoria: Crafting Lunches that Sustain and Delight"

Grilled Chicken Salad
Ingredients: Grilled chicken breast, mixed greens, cherry tomatoes, balsamic vinaigrette.
Preparation: Toss ingredients together, drizzle with vinaigrette.
Prep Time: 20 minutes.

Quinoa and Black Bean Bowl
Ingredients: Quinoa, black beans, corn, avocado.
Preparation: Mix ingredients, top with sliced avocado.
Prep Time: 15 minutes.

Salmon and Asparagus Foil Packets
Ingredients: Salmon fillet, asparagus, lemon, olive oil.
Preparation: Wrap ingredients in foil, bake.
Prep Time: 25 minutes.

Veggie Wrap with Hummus
Ingredients: Whole wheat tortilla, hummus, cucumber, bell peppers, spinach.
Preparation: Spread hummus on tortilla, add veggies, wrap it up.
Prep Time: 10 minutes.

Turkey and Avocado Lettuce Wraps

Ingredients: Turkey slices, avocado, lettuce.
Preparation: Layer turkey and avocado in lettuce leaves.
Prep Time: 10 minutes.

Whole Grain Pasta with Pesto and Cherry Tomatoes

Ingredients: Whole grain pasta, homemade pesto, cherry tomatoes.
Preparation: Cook pasta, toss with pesto and tomatoes.
Prep Time: 20 minutes.

Chickpea and Vegetable Stir-Fry

Ingredients: Chickpeas, broccoli, bell peppers, soy sauce.
Preparation: Stir-fry ingredients in a pan with soy sauce.
Prep Time: 15 minutes.

Egg Salad Lettuce Wraps

Ingredients: Hard-boiled eggs, Greek yogurt, lettuce.
Preparation: Mix eggs and yogurt, spoon onto lettuce leaves.
Prep Time: 15 minutes.

Sweet Potato and Black Bean Quesadilla
Ingredients: Sweet potato, black beans, whole wheat tortilla.
Preparation: Mash sweet potato, layer with beans, cook in a pan.
Prep Time: 20 minutes.

Mediterranean Chickpea Salad
Ingredients: Chickpeas, cherry tomatoes, cucumber, feta cheese.
Preparation: Combine ingredients, sprinkle with feta.
Prep Time: 15 minutes.

Shrimp and Broccoli Stir-Fry
Ingredients: Shrimp, broccoli, garlic, ginger.
Preparation: Stir-fry shrimp and broccoli with garlic and ginger.
Prep Time: 20 minutes.

Caprese Avocado Toast
Ingredients: Whole grain bread, tomato slices, mozzarella, avocado.
Preparation: Toast bread, top with avocado, tomato, and mozzarella.
Prep Time: 10 minutes.

Lentil and Vegetable Soup

Ingredients: Lentils, carrots, celery, vegetable broth.

Preparation: Cook ingredients in a pot with vegetable broth.

Prep Time: 30 minutes.

Tuna Salad Stuffed Bell Peppers

Ingredients: Tuna, Greek yogurt, bell peppers.

Preparation: Mix tuna and yogurt, stuff into halved bell peppers.

Prep Time: 15 minutes.

Pesto Chicken and Veggie Skewers

Ingredients: Chicken cubes, cherry tomatoes, zucchini, homemade pesto.

Preparation: Skewer ingredients, grill or bake.

Prep Time: 25 minutes.

Brown Rice Bowl with Teriyaki Tofu

Ingredients: Brown rice, tofu, teriyaki sauce, broccoli.

Preparation: Cook rice, sauté tofu with teriyaki sauce, add broccoli.

Prep Time: 25 minutes.

Greek Quinoa Salad

Ingredients: Quinoa, cucumber, olives, feta cheese.

Preparation: Mix ingredients, sprinkle with feta.

Prep Time: 15 minutes.

Turkey and Vegetable Wrap

Ingredients: Whole wheat tortilla, turkey slices, lettuce, tomato.

Preparation: Assemble ingredients into a wrap.

Prep Time: 10 minutes.

Chickpea and Avocado Salad

Ingredients: Chickpeas, avocado, cherry tomatoes, cilantro.

Preparation: Combine ingredients, garnish with cilantro.

Prep Time: 15 minutes.

Cauliflower Fried Rice

Ingredients: Cauliflower rice, peas, carrots, scrambled eggs.

Preparation: Sauté ingredients in a pan, mix with scrambled eggs.

Prep Time: 20 minutes

"Dinner Delights: Crafting Culinary Masterpieces for Heartfelt Evenings"

Baked Lemon Herb Salmon
Ingredients: Salmon fillet, lemon, herbs, olive oil.
Preparation: Season salmon, bake with lemon and herbs.
Prep Time: 20 minutes.

Vegetarian Chickpea Curry
Ingredients: Chickpeas, tomatoes, spinach, curry spices.
Preparation: Simmer ingredients in a pot with curry spices.
Prep Time: 25 minutes.

Stuffed Bell Peppers with Turkey
Ingredients: Bell peppers, ground turkey, quinoa, tomato sauce.
Preparation: Stuff peppers with turkey and quinoa, bake.
Prep Time: 30 minutes.

Baked Chicken with Roasted Vegetables
Ingredients: Chicken breasts, mixed veggies, olive oil, garlic.

Preparation: Toss chicken and veggies with olive oil, bake.
Prep Time: 25 minutes.

Whole Wheat Pasta with Tomato Basil Sauce
Ingredients: Whole wheat pasta, tomatoes, garlic, basil.
Preparation: Cook pasta, simmer tomatoes, garlic, and basil for sauce.
Prep Time: 20 minutes.

Grilled Veggie Quesadillas
Ingredients: Whole wheat tortillas, grilled veggies, cheese.
Preparation: Assemble tortillas with veggies and cheese, grill.
Prep Time: 15 minutes.

Turkey and Sweet Potato Skillet
Ingredients: Ground turkey, sweet potatoes, black beans.
Preparation: Sauté turkey, sweet potatoes, and black beans in a skillet.
Prep Time: 20 minutes.

Cauliflower Alfredo Pasta
Ingredients: Cauliflower, whole grain pasta, garlic, Parmesan.
Preparation: Blend cauliflower, garlic, and Parmesan for a creamy sauce.
Prep Time: 30 minutes.

Mango Lime Grilled Chicken
Ingredients: Chicken thighs, mango, lime, honey.
Preparation: Marinate chicken with mango, lime, and honey, grill.
Prep Time: 25 minutes.

Quinoa and Black Bean Stuffed Zucchini
Ingredients: Zucchini, quinoa, black beans, salsa.
Preparation: Scoop out zucchini, fill with quinoa and beans, bake.
Prep Time: 25 minutes.

Spaghetti Squash with Turkey Bolognese
Ingredients: Spaghetti squash, ground turkey, tomato sauce.
Preparation: Roast spaghetti squash, sauté turkey, mix with tomato sauce.
Prep Time: 30 minutes.

Lemon Garlic Shrimp Stir-Fry
Ingredients: Shrimp, broccoli, bell peppers, lemon, garlic.
Preparation: Stir-fry shrimp and veggies with lemon and garlic.
Prep Time: 20 minutes.

Chickpea and Spinach Stew
Ingredients: Chickpeas, spinach, tomatoes, cumin.
Preparation: Simmer chickpeas, spinach, and tomatoes with cumin.
Prep Time: 25 minutes.

Teriyaki Tofu and Vegetable Skewers
Ingredients: Tofu, bell peppers, zucchini, teriyaki sauce.
Preparation: Skewer tofu and veggies, grill or bake.
Prep Time: 30 minutes.

Cajun-Style Baked Tilapia
Ingredients: Tilapia fillets, Cajun spices, lemon.
Preparation: Season tilapia, bake with Cajun spices and lemon.
Prep Time: 20 minutes.

Mushroom and Spinach Stuffed Chicken
Ingredients: Chicken breasts, mushrooms, spinach, garlic.
Preparation: Sauté mushrooms and spinach, stuff into chicken, bake.
Prep Time: 30 minutes.

Sweet and Sour Turkey Meatballs
Ingredients: Ground turkey, pineapple, bell peppers, sweet and sour sauce.

Preparation: Form meatballs, bake with pineapple and peppers, drizzle with sauce.
Prep Time: 25 minutes.

Eggplant and Tomato Bake
Ingredients: Eggplant, tomatoes, mozzarella, basil.
Preparation: Layer eggplant, tomatoes, and mozzarella, bake.
Prep Time: 30 minutes.

Stir-Fried Tofu and Broccoli
Ingredients: Tofu, broccoli, soy sauce, ginger.
Preparation: Stir-fry tofu and broccoli with soy sauce and ginger.
Prep Time: 20 minutes.

Sesame Ginger Glazed Salmon
Ingredients: Salmon fillet, sesame ginger glaze, green onions.
Preparation: Brush salmon with glaze, bake, sprinkle with green onions.
Prep Time: 25 minutes.

Snacks and Appetizers

"Cravings Conquered: Indulging in Snacks and Sweets, the Heart-Healthy Way"

Greek Yogurt and Berry Parfait
Ingredients: Greek yogurt, mixed berries, granola.
Preparation: Layer yogurt, berries, and granola.
Prep Time: 5 minutes.

Homemade Hummus with Veggie Sticks
Ingredients: Chickpeas, tahini, olive oil, carrot and cucumber sticks.
Preparation: Blend chickpeas, tahini, and olive oil, served with veggie sticks.
Prep Time: 10 minutes.

Avocado and Tomato Salsa
Ingredients: Avocado, tomatoes, onion, cilantro.
Preparation: Dice ingredients, mix together.
Prep Time: 15 minutes.

Crispy Kale Chips
Ingredients: Kale leaves, olive oil, sea salt.
Preparation: Toss kale in oil, bake until crispy.
Prep Time: 15 minutes.

Whole Grain Crackers with Smoked Salmon

Ingredients: Whole grain crackers, smoked salmon, cream cheese.

Preparation: Spread cream cheese on crackers, top with smoked salmon.

Prep Time: 10 minutes.

Banana and Almond Butter Bites

Ingredients: Banana slices, almond butter, chia seeds.

Preparation: Spread almond butter on banana slices, sprinkle with chia seeds.

Prep Time: 5 minutes.

Edamame and Sea Salt Pods

Ingredients: Edamame pods, sea salt.

Preparation: Boil edamame, sprinkle with sea salt.

Prep Time: 10 minutes.

Mango Salsa with Baked Pita Chips

Ingredients: Mango, red onion, lime, whole wheat pita.

Preparation: Dice ingredients for salsa, bake pita into chips.

Prep Time: 20 minutes.

Cottage Cheese and Pineapple Skewers

Ingredients: Cottage cheese, pineapple chunks.
Preparation: Skewer cottage cheese and pineapple.
Prep Time: 10 minutes.

Roasted Red Pepper and Walnut Dip

Ingredients: Roasted red peppers, walnuts, garlic.
Preparation: Blend ingredients into a dip.
Prep Time: 15 minutes.

Sweet Potato Toast with Avocado

Ingredients: Sweet potato slices, avocado, cherry tomatoes.
Preparation: Toast sweet potato slices, top with mashed avocado and tomatoes.
Prep Time: 20 minutes.

Turkey and Cheese Roll-Ups

Ingredients: Turkey slices, cheese, whole grain tortilla.
Preparation: Layer turkey and cheese on tortilla, roll it up.
Prep Time: 10 minutes.

Apple Slices with Almond Butter

Ingredients: Apple slices, almond butter.
Preparation: Spread almond butter on apple slices.
Prep Time: 5 minutes.

Caprese Skewers
Ingredients: Cherry tomatoes, mozzarella balls, basil leaves.
Preparation: Skewer tomatoes, mozzarella, and basil.
Prep Time: 10 minutes.

Mixed Nuts and Dried Fruit Bowl
Ingredients: Mixed nuts, dried fruit.
Preparation: Combine nuts and dried fruit in a bowl.
Prep Time: 5 minutes.

Sliced Cucumber with Tzatziki
Ingredients: Cucumber slices, tzatziki sauce.
Preparation: Dip cucumber slices in tzatziki.
Prep Time: 10 minutes.

Trail Mix Popcorn
Ingredients: Popcorn, almonds, dried cranberries.
Preparation: Mix popcorn with almonds and cranberries.
Prep Time: 15 minutes.

Stuffed Cherry Tomatoes with Goat Cheese
Ingredients: Cherry tomatoes, goat cheese, balsamic glaze.
Preparation: Hollow out tomatoes, fill with goat cheese, drizzle with balsamic glaze.
Prep Time: 15 minutes.

Spiced Roasted Chickpeas
Ingredients: Chickpeas, olive oil, cumin.
Preparation: Toss chickpeas in oil and cumin, roast until crispy.
Prep Time: 25 minutes.

Yogurt-Dipped Strawberries
Ingredients: Strawberries, Greek yogurt.
Preparation: Dip strawberries in Greek yogurt.
Prep Time: 10 minutes.

Sweet Desserts

Berry and Yogurt Parfait
Ingredients: Mixed berries, Greek yogurt, honey.
Preparation: Layer berries and yogurt, drizzle with honey.
Prep Time: 10 minutes.

Dark Chocolate-Dipped Strawberries
Ingredients: Strawberries, dark chocolate.
Preparation: Melt chocolate, dip strawberries, let them cool.
Prep Time: 15 minutes.

Banana and Almond Butter Ice Cream
Ingredients: Frozen bananas, almond butter.
Preparation: Blend frozen bananas with almond butter until creamy.
Prep Time: 5 minutes.

Chia Seed Pudding with Mango
Ingredients: Chia seeds, almond milk, mango.
Preparation: Mix chia seeds and almond milk, refrigerate, top with mango.
Prep Time: 5 minutes (plus chilling time).

Baked Apples with Cinnamon
Ingredients: Apples, cinnamon, a touch of honey.
Preparation: Core apples, sprinkle with cinnamon, bake.
Prep Time: 20 minutes.

Frozen Blueberry Yogurt Bites
Ingredients: Blueberries, Greek yogurt.
Preparation: Dip blueberries in yogurt, freeze.
Prep Time: 10 minutes (plus freezing time).

Avocado Chocolate Mousse
Ingredients: Avocado, cocoa powder, honey.
Preparation: Blend avocado, cocoa powder, and honey until smooth.
Prep Time: 10 minutes.

Peach and Almond Crumble
Ingredients: Peaches, almonds, oats.
Preparation: Mix sliced peaches with crushed almonds and oats, bake.
Prep Time: 25 minutes.

Raspberry Oat Bars
Ingredients: Oats, raspberries, almond butter.
Preparation: Mix oats and almond butter, layer with raspberries, bake.
Prep Time: 20 minutes.

Coconut and Berry Chia Popsicles
Ingredients: Coconut milk, mixed berries, chia seeds.
Preparation: Mix ingredients, pour into popsicle molds, freeze.
Prep Time: 10 minutes (plus freezing time).

Apple Cinnamon Oatmeal Cookies
Ingredients: Rolled oats, apples, cinnamon.
Preparation: Mix oats, apples, and cinnamon, bake into cookies.
Prep Time: 15 minutes.

Strawberry and Almond Sorbet
Ingredients: Strawberries, almond milk, a touch of honey.
Preparation: Blend strawberries, almond milk, and honey, freeze.
Prep Time: 10 minutes (plus freezing time).

Vanilla and Berry Smoothie Bowl
Ingredients: Mixed berries, almond milk, vanilla extract.
Preparation: Blend berries, almond milk, and vanilla, pour into a bowl.

Prep Time: 5 minutes.

Cinnamon Baked Pears

Ingredients: Pears, cinnamon, a drizzle of maple syrup.

Preparation: Slice pears, sprinkle with cinnamon, bake.

Prep Time: 15 minutes.

Cherry and Almond Energy Bites

Ingredients: Dried cherries, almonds, dates.

Preparation: Blend ingredients, roll into bite-sized balls.

Prep Time: 15 minutes.

Chocolate Banana Nice Cream

Ingredients: Frozen bananas, cocoa powder.

Preparation: Blend frozen bananas with cocoa powder until creamy.

Prep Time: 5 minutes.

Oat and Berry Breakfast Bars

Ingredients: Oats, mixed berries, a touch of honey.

Preparation: Mix oats and berries, bake into bars.

Prep Time: 20 minutes.

Pineapple Coconut Chia Pudding
Ingredients: Chia seeds, coconut milk, diced pineapple.
Preparation: Mix chia seeds with coconut milk, refrigerate, top with pineapple.
Prep Time: 5 minutes (plus chilling time).

Mango and Lime Sorbet
Ingredients: Mango, lime juice, a touch of agave nectar.
Preparation: Blend mango, lime juice, and agave, freeze.
Prep Time: 10 minutes (plus freezing time).

Almond Butter and Banana Sandwiches
Ingredients: Whole grain bread, almond butter, banana slices.
Preparation: Spread almond butter on bread, add banana slices, make a sandwich.
Prep Time: 5 minutes.

Berry Blast Smoothie
Ingredients: Mixed berries, Greek yogurt, almond milk.
Preparation: Blend berries, yogurt, and almond milk until smooth.
Prep Time: 5 minutes.

Green Goodness Detox Drink
Ingredients: Spinach, cucumber, apple, lemon.
Preparation: Juice spinach, cucumber, apple, and lemon.
Prep Time: 10 minutes.

Tropical Paradise Smoothie
Ingredients: Pineapple, mango, coconut water.
Preparation: Blend pineapple, mango, and coconut water.
Prep Time: 5 minutes.

Heart-Healthy Green Tea
Ingredients: Green tea, mint leaves, honey.
Preparation: Brew green tea, add mint leaves and honey.
Prep Time: 5 minutes.

Cucumber Mint Cooler
Ingredients: Cucumber, mint, lime, sparkling water.
Preparation: Muddle cucumber and mint, add lime, top with sparkling water.
Prep Time: 10 minutes.

Protein-Packed Almond Butter Smoothie
Ingredients: Banana, almond butter, almond milk, protein powder.
Preparation: Blend banana, almond butter, almond milk, and protein powder.
Prep Time: 5 minutes.

Refreshing Watermelon Slush
Ingredients: Watermelon, lime, ice.
Preparation: Blend watermelon and lime with ice.
Prep Time: 5 minutes.

Chia Seed and Berry Hydration
Ingredients: Chia seeds, mixed berries, coconut water.
Preparation: Mix chia seeds, berries, and coconut water.
Prep Time: 10 minutes (plus soaking time).

Pomegranate Punch

Ingredients: Pomegranate juice, sparkling water, lime.

Preparation: Mix pomegranate juice with sparkling water, add lime.

Prep Time: 5 minutes.

Strawberry Banana Oat Smoothie

Ingredients: Strawberries, banana, oats, almond milk.

Preparation: Blend strawberries, banana, oats, and almond milk.

Prep Time: 5 minutes.

Ginger Lemon Turmeric Elixir

Ingredients: Ginger, lemon, turmeric, honey.

Preparation: Juice ginger, lemon, and turmeric, add honey.

Prep Time: 10 minutes.

Minty Blueberry Lemonade

Ingredients: Blueberries, mint, lemon, water.

Preparation: Muddle blueberries and mint, add lemon and water.

Prep Time: 10 minutes.

Creamy Avocado Spinach Smoothie
Ingredients: Avocado, spinach, banana, coconut milk.
Preparation: Blend avocado, spinach, banana, and coconut milk.
Prep Time: 5 minutes.

Cranberry Orange Sparkler
Ingredients: Cranberry juice, orange slices, sparkling water.
Preparation: Mix cranberry juice with sparkling water, add orange slices.
Prep Time: 5 minutes.

Anti-Inflammatory Cherry Turmeric Smoothie
Ingredients: Cherries, turmeric, Greek yogurt, almond milk.
Preparation: Blend cherries, turmeric, yogurt, and almond milk.
Prep Time: 5 minutes.

Coconut Pineapple Refresher
Ingredients: Coconut water, pineapple, mint.
Preparation: Blend coconut water, pineapple, and mint.
Prep Time: 5 minutes.

Berry-Licious Iced Tea

Ingredients: Mixed berries, black tea, honey.
Preparation: Brew black tea, add mixed berries and honey, chill.
Prep Time: 10 minutes.

Chocolate Banana Smoothie

Ingredients: Banana, cocoa powder, almond milk, honey.
Preparation: Blend banana, cocoa powder, almond milk, and honey.
Prep Time: 5 minutes.

Golden Milk Latte

Ingredients: Turmeric, cinnamon, ginger, almond milk.
Preparation: Mix turmeric, cinnamon, and ginger into almond milk, warm.
Prep Time: 10 minutes.

Raspberry Lemon Basil Infused Water

Ingredients: Raspberries, lemon slices, basil leaves.
Preparation: Infuse water with raspberries, lemon, and basil.
Prep Time: 5 minutes.

CONCLUSION

"Your Heart, Your Symphony: The Finale of Your AFib Diet Journey"

As we draw the curtains on this culinary and wellness odyssey, let's take a moment to savor the enriching lessons and delectable recipes that have adorned our journey. Your commitment to a heart-healthy lifestyle has been a symphony, each chapter a note in the melody of your well-being. Here's a heartfelt recap and a gentle nudge to continue your harmonious journey.

Recap of Key Lessons:
Understanding AFib: We unraveled the intricacies of Atrial Fibrillation, paving the way for informed choices in managing and nurturing your heart.

The Science of Nutrition and Heart Health: Delved into the essential nutrients and scientific foundations that underpin a heart-healthy diet, creating a tapestry of wellness on your plate.

Stocking Your Heart-Healthy Kitchen: Equipped you with the knowledge to select ingredients that nourish and fortify your heart, transforming your kitchen into a sanctuary of health.

Delicious Breakfasts, Lunches, Dinners, Snacks, and Desserts: Presented a palette of mouthwatering recipes, marrying flavor with heart health in each culinary creation.

Lifestyle Tips for a Heart-Happy Life: Stepped beyond the plate to explore holistic habits, embracing exercise, stress management, and restful sleep as essential notes in the symphony of heart well-being.

Your journey doesn't conclude here; it merely transforms into the next beautiful movement. As you stand at the threshold of a heart-happy future, let encouragement be your steadfast companion. Every wholesome meal, every mindful breath, and every step taken in the direction of heart health is a testament to your resilience and commitment.

Continue to savor the joy of crafting heart-healthy masterpieces in your kitchen. Let each meal be a celebration of life, a declaration that your heart deserves nothing less than the best. Remember, this journey is uniquely yours, and each choice you make is a brushstroke on the canvas of your vibrant heart.

14 DAYS MEAL PLAN

Day 1:
Breakfast: Berry Overnight Oats
Ingredients: Rolled oats, almond milk, mixed berries, chia seeds.
Preparation: Mix oats, almond milk, berries, and chia seeds in a jar, refrigerate overnight.
Prep Time: 5 minutes (plus overnight soaking).

Lunch: Grilled Chicken Salad
Ingredients: Grilled chicken breast, mixed greens, cherry tomatoes, cucumber, olive oil, balsamic vinegar.
Preparation: Toss grilled chicken and veggies, drizzle with olive oil and balsamic vinegar.
Prep Time: 20 minutes.

Dinner: Baked Salmon with Quinoa
Ingredients: Salmon fillet, quinoa, lemon, garlic, olive oil.
Preparation: Season salmon, bake with quinoa, lemon, and garlic.
Prep Time: 30 minutes.

Day 2:
Breakfast: Green Smoothie
Ingredients: Spinach, banana, pineapple, Greek yogurt, almond milk.

Preparation: Blend spinach, banana, pineapple, yogurt, and almond milk.
Prep Time: 5 minutes.

Lunch: Turkey and Avocado Wrap

Ingredients: Whole grain wrap, sliced turkey, avocado, lettuce, tomato.
Preparation: Assemble ingredients in a wrap.
Prep Time: 10 minutes.

Dinner: Veggie Stir-Fry with Brown Rice

Ingredients: Mixed vegetables, tofu, soy sauce, brown rice.
Preparation: Stir-fry veggies and tofu, add soy sauce, serve over brown rice.
Prep Time: 25 minutes.

Day 3:

Breakfast: Greek Yogurt Parfait

Ingredients: Greek yogurt, granola, mixed berries, honey.
Preparation: Layer yogurt, granola, berries, and honey.
Prep Time: 5 minutes.

Lunch: Quinoa Salad with Chickpeas

Ingredients: Quinoa, chickpeas, cucumber, feta cheese, olive oil, lemon.
Preparation: Mix cooked quinoa, chickpeas, cucumber, feta, olive oil, and lemon.
Prep Time: 15 minutes.

Dinner: Baked Cod with Sweet Potato
Ingredients: Cod fillet, sweet potato, olive oil, lemon, thyme.
Preparation: Season cod, bake with sweet potato, olive oil, lemon, and thyme.
Prep Time: 30 minutes.

Day 4:
Breakfast: Banana Almond Butter Smoothie
Ingredients: Banana, almond butter, almond milk, oats.
Preparation: Blend banana, almond butter, almond milk, and oats.
Prep Time: 5 minutes.

Lunch: Lentil Soup
Ingredients: Lentils, carrots, celery, onion, vegetable broth.
Preparation: Simmer lentils, carrots, celery, and onion in vegetable broth.
Prep Time: 30 minutes.

Dinner: Grilled Shrimp with Quinoa Salad
Ingredients: Shrimp, quinoa, cherry tomatoes, avocado, lime, cilantro.
Preparation: Grill shrimp, mix with quinoa, tomatoes, avocado, lime, and cilantro.
Prep Time: 25 minutes.

Day 5:

Breakfast: Chia Seed Pudding with Berries
Ingredients: Chia seeds, almond milk, mixed berries.
Preparation: Mix chia seeds and almond milk, refrigerate, top with berries.
Prep Time: 5 minutes (plus chilling time).

Lunch: Caprese Salad
Ingredients: Tomatoes, mozzarella, basil, olive oil, balsamic vinegar.
Preparation: Arrange sliced tomatoes, mozzarella, and basil, drizzle with olive oil and balsamic vinegar.
Prep Time: 10 minutes.

Dinner: Baked Chicken with Roasted Vegetables
Ingredients: Chicken breasts, mixed vegetables, olive oil, garlic.
Preparation: Toss chicken and veggies with olive oil, bake.
Prep Time: 25 minutes.

Day 6:

Breakfast: Spinach and Mushroom Omelette
Ingredients: Eggs, spinach, mushrooms, feta cheese.
Preparation: Whisk eggs, sauté spinach and mushrooms, make an omelette with feta.
Prep Time: 15 minutes.

Lunch: Chickpea and Avocado Salad
Ingredients: Chickpeas, avocado, cherry tomatoes, red onion, lemon, olive oil.
Preparation: Mix chickpeas, avocado, tomatoes, and onion, drizzle with lemon and olive oil.
Prep Time: 10 minutes.

Dinner: Teriyaki Tofu Stir-Fry with Brown Rice
Ingredients: Tofu, broccoli, bell peppers, teriyaki sauce, brown rice.
Preparation: Stir-fry tofu and veggies, add teriyaki sauce, serve over brown rice.
Prep Time: 25 minutes.

Day 7:
Breakfast: Blueberry Banana Pancakes
Ingredients: Whole wheat flour, blueberries, banana, almond milk.
Preparation: Mix flour, blueberries, banana, and almond milk, cook as pancakes.
Prep Time: 20 minutes.

Lunch: Quinoa and Black Bean Bowl
Ingredients: Quinoa, black beans, corn, avocado, salsa.
Preparation: Combine cooked quinoa, black beans, corn, and avocado, top with salsa.
Prep Time: 15 minutes.

Dinner: Lemon Garlic Salmon with Asparagus
Ingredients: Salmon fillet, asparagus, lemon, garlic, olive oil.
Preparation: Season salmon and asparagus with lemon, garlic, and olive oil, bake.
Prep Time: 30 minutes.

Day 8:
Breakfast: Peach and Almond Butter Toast
Ingredients: Whole grain bread, peach slices, almond butter.
Preparation: Toast bread, spread almond butter, top with peach slices.
Prep Time: 10 minutes.

Lunch: Mediterranean Quinoa Salad
Ingredients: Quinoa, cherry tomatoes, cucumber, olives, feta cheese, olive oil.
Preparation: Mix cooked quinoa, tomatoes, cucumber, olives, feta, and olive oil.
Prep Time: 15 minutes.

Dinner: Grilled Vegetable and Chicken Skewers
Ingredients: Chicken breast, bell peppers, zucchini, cherry tomatoes, balsamic glaze.
Preparation: Thread chicken and veggies on skewers, grill, drizzle with balsamic glaze.
Prep Time: 25 minutes.

Day 9:
Breakfast: Mango Coconut Chia Pudding
Ingredients: Chia seeds, coconut milk, mango chunks.
Preparation: Mix chia seeds and coconut milk, refrigerate, top with mango.
Prep Time: 5 minutes (plus chilling time).

Lunch: Turkey and Quinoa Stuffed Peppers
Ingredients: Ground turkey, quinoa, bell peppers, tomatoes, black beans.
Preparation: Cook turkey and quinoa, stuff into halved bell peppers, bake.
Prep Time: 30 minutes.

Dinner: Shrimp and Broccoli Stir-Fry with Cauliflower Rice
Ingredients: Shrimp, broccoli, cauliflower rice, soy sauce.
Preparation: Stir-fry shrimp and broccoli, serve over cauliflower rice with soy sauce.
Prep Time: 20 minutes.

Day 10:
Breakfast: Apple Cinnamon Chia Seed Pudding
Ingredients: Chia seeds, almond milk, apple slices, cinnamon.
Preparation: Mix chia seeds and almond milk, refrigerate, top with apple slices and cinnamon.
Prep Time: 5 minutes (plus chilling time).

Lunch: Avocado and Chickpea Wrap

Ingredients: Whole grain wrap, avocado, chickpeas, lettuce, salsa.

Preparation: Mash chickpeas and avocado, spread in a wrap with lettuce and salsa.

Prep Time: 10 minutes.

Dinner: Baked Cod with Mango Salsa

Ingredients: Cod fillet, mango, red onion, cilantro, lime.

Preparation: Season cod, bake, top with mango salsa.

Prep Time: 25 minutes.

Day 11:

Breakfast: Raspberry Coconut Smoothie Bowl

Ingredients: Raspberries, coconut milk, banana, shredded coconut.

Preparation: Blend raspberries, coconut milk, and banana, pour into a bowl, top with shredded coconut.

Prep Time: 10 minutes.

Lunch: Spinach and Feta Stuffed Chicken Breast

Ingredients: Chicken breast, spinach, feta cheese, garlic.

Preparation: Stuff chicken breast with sautéed spinach, feta, and garlic, bake.

Prep Time: 30 minutes.

Dinner: Lentil and Vegetable Curry with Brown Rice
Ingredients: Lentils, mixed vegetables, curry sauce, brown rice.
Preparation: Cook lentils and veggies in curry sauce, serve over brown rice.
Prep Time: 25 minutes.

Day 12:
Breakfast: Peanut Butter Banana Smoothie
Ingredients: Banana, peanut butter, almond milk, oats.
Preparation: Blend banana, peanut butter, almond milk, and oats.
Prep Time: 5 minutes.

Lunch: Mediterranean Chickpea Wrap
Ingredients: Whole grain wrap, chickpeas, cherry tomatoes, cucumber, hummus.
Preparation: Assemble ingredients in a wrap with a spread of hummus.
Prep Time: 10 minutes.

Dinner: Grilled Tofu Skewers with Quinoa
Ingredients: Tofu, bell peppers, red onion, quinoa, balsamic glaze.
Preparation: Thread tofu and veggies on skewers, grill, serve over quinoa with balsamic glaze.
Prep Time: 25 minutes.

Day 13:

Breakfast: Blueberry Almond Butter Toast
Ingredients: Whole grain bread, blueberries, almond butter.
Preparation: Toast bread, spread almond butter, top with blueberries.
Prep Time: 10 minutes.

Lunch: Caprese Quinoa Salad
Ingredients: Quinoa, cherry tomatoes, mozzarella, basil, balsamic glaze.
Preparation: Mix cooked quinoa, tomatoes, mozzarella, and basil, drizzle with balsamic glaze.
Prep Time: 15 minutes.

Dinner: Lemon Herb Chicken with Sweet Potato
Ingredients: Chicken thighs, sweet potato, lemon, thyme, rosemary.
Preparation: Season chicken thighs and sweet potato with lemon, thyme, and rosemary, bake.
Prep Time: 30 minutes.

Day 14:

Breakfast: Banana Walnut Overnight Oats
Ingredients: Rolled oats, almond milk, banana slices, walnuts.
Preparation: Mix oats, almond milk, banana slices, and walnuts in a jar, refrigerate overnight.
Prep Time: 5 minutes (plus overnight soaking).

Lunch: Quinoa and Black Bean Stuffed Bell Peppers

Ingredients: Quinoa, black beans, bell peppers, salsa.

Preparation: Cook quinoa and black beans, stuff into halved bell peppers, top with salsa.

Prep Time: 30 minutes.

Dinner: Garlic Herb Baked Salmon with Asparagus

Ingredients: Salmon fillet, asparagus, garlic, herbs, olive oil.

Preparation: Season salmon and asparagus with garlic, herbs, and olive oil, bake.

Prep Time: 30 minutes.

Shopping list

Fruits:

1. Blueberries
2. Strawberries
3. Raspberries
4. Bananas
5. Mango
6. Apples
7. Pears
8. Peaches
9. Oranges
10. Lemons
11. Avocado
12. Watermelon

13. Pineapple

Vegetables:
1. Spinach
2. Kale
3. Broccoli
4. Cauliflower
5. Bell peppers (assorted colors)
6. Zucchini
7. Carrots
8. Cucumber
9. Tomatoes
10. Sweet potatoes
11. Asparagus
12. Red onion
13. Garlic

Leafy Greens:
1. Romaine lettuce
2. Mixed salad greens
3. Arugula
4. Swiss chard

Proteins:
1. Salmon fillets
2. Cod fillets
3. Shrimp
4. Chicken breasts
5. Turkey slices
6. Tofu
7. Lentils

8. Chickpeas
9. Black beans

Dairy and Alternatives:
1. Greek yogurt
2. Feta cheese
3. Mozzarella cheese
4. Almond milk
5. Coconut milk

Grains and Carbs:
1. Quinoa
2. Brown rice
3. Whole wheat flour
4. Rolled oats
5. Whole grain bread
6. Whole grain wraps

Nuts and Seeds:
1. Almonds
2. Walnuts
3. Chia seeds
4. Flaxseeds

Nut Butters:
1. Almond butter
2. Peanut butter
3. Oils and Condiments:
4. Olive oil
5. Avocado oil

6. Balsamic vinegar
7. Soy sauce
8. Hummus

Herbs and Spices:
1. Basil
2. Cilantro
3. Thyme
4. Rosemary
5. Mint
6. Cinnamon
7. Turmeric
8. Ginger

Sweeteners:
1. Honey
2. Agave nectar
3. Frozen Section:
4. Mixed berries (frozen)
5. Mango chunks (frozen)
6. Spinach (frozen)

Seafood (if fresh):
1. Scallops
2. Mussels

Beverages:
1. Green tea
2. Herbal tea

Canned Goods:
1. Canned tuna (in water)
2. Canned salmon

3. Diced tomatoes (no added salt)
4. Tomato sauce (no added sugar)

Condiments and Sauces:
1. Salsa (fresh or jarred)
2. Mustard
3. Hot sauce

Alternative Flours:
1. Almond flour
2. Coconut flour

Alternative Sweeteners:
1. Stevia

Whole Grains:
2. Barley
3. Farro

Dairy Alternatives:
1. Soy milk
2. Oat milk

Miscellaneous:
1. Vine-ripened tomatoes
2. Quinoa pasta
3. Coconut water
4. Canned chickpeas
5. Whole-grain tortillas
6. Dark chocolate (70% cocoa or higher)
7. Nutritional yeast
8. Vegetable broth (low-sodium)